YOUR KNOWLEDGE HAS VALUE

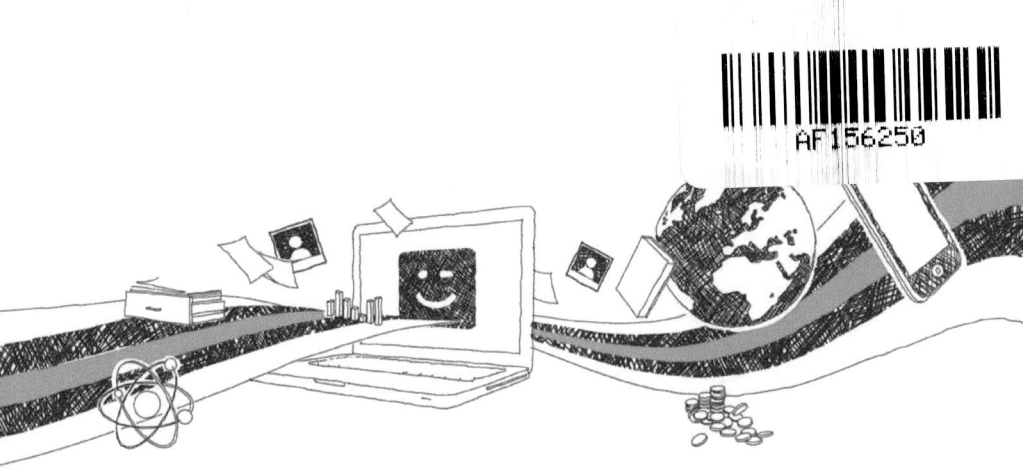

AF156250

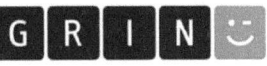

Junaid Javaid

Healthcare tourism opportunities for India

GRIN Publishing

Bibliographic information published by the German National Library:

The German National Library lists this publication in the National Bibliography; detailed bibliographic data are available on the Internet at http://dnb.dnb.de .

Imprint:

Copyright © 2013 GRIN Verlag GmbH
Print and binding: Books on Demand GmbH, Norderstedt Germany
ISBN: 978-3-656-73429-1

This book at GRIN:

http://www.grin.com/en/e-book/279772/healthcare-tourism-opportunities-for-india

GRIN - Your knowledge has value

Since its foundation in 1998, GRIN has specialized in publishing academic texts by students, college teachers and other academics as e-book and printed book. The website www.grin.com is an ideal platform for presenting term papers, final papers, scientific essays, dissertations and specialist books.

Visit us on the internet:

http://www.grin.com/

http://www.facebook.com/grincom

http://www.twitter.com/grin_com

HEALTHCARE TOURISM OPPRTUNITIES FOR INDIA

FINAL REPORT

SHR060-6: THEORY INTO PRACTICE

WRITTEN & SUBMITTED BY:
   JUNAID JAVAID

COURSE TITLE:
   MASTER OF BUSINESS ADMINISTRATION IN HEALTHCARE & HOSPITAL MANAGEMENT

DATE OF SUBMISSION:
   18-MAY-2013

Table of Contents

Executive Summary

This report is written on the topic of 'Healthcare Tourism Opportunities for India'. The scope of this report is broad as it incorporates the case studies of five major players in Indian healthcare tourism sector. It has been observed that Healthcare Tourism and Medical Tourism are interchangeable terms. In general, there are two main causes (developed countries' increasing cost of healthcare services and their overburdened healthcare infrastructure) that have resulted in enhancing the demand for healthcare tourism. Medical Malpractices Insurance is the major for increasing the healthcare cost in developed countries. Commonly, medical malpractice insurance is considered as major aspect for increasing the cost of medical treatment, widening the delay in the waitlist and also enhancing the movement of medical professionals from one region to another. India has competitive edge in the healthcare tourism because of certain characteristics: healthcare professional availability, low-cost medical treatment, enhancing popularity of its traditional wellness systems and country's existing reputation for treat of relatively advance healthcare segments (such as organ transplant, cardio-vascular surgery and eye surgery/ By reviewing all the case studies, it has been analysed that there are certain general practices that are being pursued by major healthcare service providers in India. It includes updation and utilisation of advanced technology & medical facilities, consistent healthcare education, research in medical sciences and the approach of skill development. It has been discovered that there are certain opportunities (Increasing cost of healthcare in developed countries, language proficiency of Indians, Indian healthcare institutions' success rate, delay in waiting time, Indian healthcare institutions' success rate and spillover effects) that could be exploited by the Indian medical institutions that are intended on providing medical services to foreign medical tourists. However, it has been determined that Indian medical tourism sector has been some of the challenges (Indian government's low spending on Healthcare sector, lack of International Accreditation, transplantation law, shortage of hotel accommodation and inadequate malpractices law) that could have negative impact on the growth rate of this sector. It has been recommended that the strategies currently adopted by major players of Indian medical tourism sector have helped its country to emerge as favourite healthcare destination for foreign medical tourists.

Section-1: Background Context and Aims & Objectives

1.1. Background Context

From the economics perspective, more often the countries' wealth estimates through the form of health services provided to their citizen. It has been observed that almost all countries are in the pursuit of providing sustainable healthcare solutions to its population. Corresponding, improvements in the healthcare sector is perceived as more than the availability of hospitals, doctors and medicines (James, 1989). However, improvement in the healthcare happens as a result of promotion of healthcare consciousness which is normally done through various marketing activities that would be suitable for multiple sections (elders, youth and children) of given society. From this point of view, traditional healthcare systems of India (specifically Yoga and Ayurveda) are regarded as a conception of spiritual healings that are very famous and effective among national and international tourists (George & Swamy, 2012).

Generally, a person is called as healthcare tourist if he/she travels from one country to another for undergoing medical treatment (Jagyasi, 2011). While, this definition of healthcare tourist has neglected certain persons who used to travel to another country for exploring, enjoying and rejuvenating[1] their minds and body without undertaking any sort of medical treatment. Specifically, the flow of tourists is far more in an absolute term along with the profits generated through this aspect if one country would strongly consider this aspect. It has been determined that there are many tourist attractions located in India that have healing abilities and are relatedly capable of offering life rewarding experiences. Himalayan mountain ranges are in the northern part hence the country's southern region (long coastline) is surrounded by sea. Additionally, country has many historical sites, landscapes, royal cities, serene mountain retreats and clean beaches. India also have different cultures which meant that festivals are used to be held throughout all the year. And in this way people from other countries would enjoy and rejuvenate themselves (REDDY, 2013).

---

[1] Traveling to places like mountains, sea-side, forests, riverbeds, valleys, plains or historic monuments located in other countries.

Main aim of this research report is to review global medical tourism industry and to analyse the demand for Indian medical care institution from the perspective of medical tourists. Relatedly, it significant to signify medical tourism solutions exist in India. It will importantly take account of exclusiveness of Indian healthcare institutions concentrating on providing medical care solutions to their medical tourists located in foreign countries.

Moreover, it has been contended that Healthcare Tourism and Medical Tourism are interchangeable terms. The concept called as medical tourism is basically from the practice where people belong to developed countries are traveling to the developing countries for the purpose of receiving long range of medical services significantly because of increasing cost of medical services available in their native countries (Stolley & Watson, 2012). Relatedly, complicated treatment procedures are also determined as associated reason. In short, medical tourism is referred as cost effective provision for purpose of providing private medical services in combination with the tourism sector prominently for patients requiring surgical and associated treatment. However, healthcare tourism is described in a broader prospect where the patients are desiring to travel aboard with the motive of overall wellness with any elective or urgent medical procedures (Connell, 2011).

Basically, there are two major forms of healthcare solutions (traditional and modern systems of medicine). It has been learnt that the traditional systems originated from long period of time in almost all countries this happened as an outcome of competitive environment which had gone through variation in term of providing healing solutions (Mal, 2010). However, some of them are scientific based and others are realised to be based on providing healing solutions (spiritual or faith healing). And it has been found out that such form of healing solutions are existing in some countries (India, Nepal, Malaysia and Philippines). Correspondingly, it has been discovered that such kind of travel segment is regarded as fastest growing segments especially in the global tourism industry (Mudur, 2004).

It has been believed that healthcare tourism has many distinctive characteristics. The most vital feature is that it is not an impulsive activity (Woodward et al., 2001). And it used to be offered in the form of attractive features that would be enough for targeting foreign medical tourists. Second attribute is that it is not directly related with the aspect of willingness to spend and this feature thus incorporate certain tourists who are not willing to spend but their health conditions intend them to travel & spend (Gautam, 2008). Third feature is that healthcare tourism is not a seasonal sector, this has been supported with a fact that the duration of stay under the provision of healthcare tourism is considerably longer than holiday or conventional corporate travel (Langenbrunner et al., 2011). Last characteristic is that it is not a onetime business which has been proved with an aspect that successful medical treatment is directly linked with satisfactory services that in turn increase the chances of getting repeat business.

1.2. Motivation

The motivation behind choosing this topic is my interest and existing knowledge about the healthcare tourism sector. As I'm from India and my country is emerging as only big player in the given field. This aspect of medical care tourism not only intended to increase the profits of these service providers but also have generated a lot of working opportunity. And all in all, these all things are making positive impact on our country's GDP and also has enhance the level of healthcare services provided at local level as well. So, the reason behind outlining all of these facts is that I would want to get employed in the given sector and then would run my own medical tourism institution.

1.3. Aim & Objectives

The core objective of this report is to signify certain opportunities and challenges for the Health Service Providers in India from the global perspective. Additionally, other related objectives have been listed below:

- To examine the tourism scenario in World and Indian healthcare market.
- To analyse the demand for healthcare tourism in the World.
- To identify the healthcare & tourism solutions existing in India in order to cater the demand for Healthcare Tourism.
- To consider the exclusiveness of India in regard to the different segments within the tourism & healthcare solutions.

1.4. Methods

This theory into practice report will be based on secondary research method. And the case study approach will be adopted in order to create between literature review and case study sections. In this manner, it would enable to accomplish certain objectives that have been listed above.

Section-2: Literature Review

2.1. World's Healthcare Tourism Market

The revenue generated by world's healthcare tourism market is more than $40 billion. And this market is growing at a rate of 20%. In 2007, the size of the market was around $150 billion and it has been predicted to be double by the end of 2015 (Gautam, 2008). From broader perspective, there are massive opportunities incorporated in this market.

2.2. Demand Drivers

In general, there are two main causes (developed countries' increasing cost of healthcare services and their overburdened healthcare infrastructure) that have resulted in enhancing the demand for healthcare tourism (Hall, 2013). On other hand, improvement in developing countries healthcare systems & technologies are the contributing factor for the growth of healthcare tourism. It has been observed the ratio of individual without insurance (specifically below the age of 65) has incremented from 29.8 million in 1984 to approximately 41.6 million in 2004 (Shah, 2006). And out of these uninsured persons more than 50% belongs to the Asian races. Therefore, shortcoming of vibrant procedures for defining & managing waitlists is the prominent factor that have negative impact on the length of waitlists. Correspondingly, insufficient specialists' supplies, operating rooms, surgeons, technology and para-medical staff are also determined as main reasons that intended foreign patients to come to developing countries and acquire services of equivalent but at relatively lower cost (Sarkar, 2009).

2.3. Medical Malpractices Insurance

Medical Malpractices Insurance is the major for increasing the healthcare cost in developed countries. This insurance normally covers the liability claims of doctors & other professional in the specified field and it generally occurs from their patients' treatment. Relatedly, it also occurs during the time when a physician unable to treat in a proper manner. Commonly, medical malpractice insurance is considered as major aspect for increasing the cost of medical treatment, widening the delay in the waitlist and also enhancing the movement of medical professionals from one region to another (MIRRER-SINGER, 2007). Hence it has been seen that the increment in the cost of medical treatment also directs towards unaffordable premium in relation to insurance by individuals and thus put large amount of people out from the bracket of health insurance coverage (Vick, 2012).

Additionally, it has been believed that the second major cause of increasing of medical treatment cost is the sudden increase of premium expense which used to be pursued through medical malpractice insurance. It has been observed that the insurance have begun to increase the premium for medical malpractice insurance the with the increase in the volume of claims (Hartwig & Wilkinson, 2003) It has been found out the underwriting losses in relation to malpractice insurance had dramatically increased from $230 million in 1990 to $3billion after 11 years in United States.

2.4. Major Countries in Healthcare Tourism

It has been analysed that there are certain countries (Malaysia, Thailand, Singapore, China, Philippines, Cuba, South Africa, Jordan and India) are battling hard for the capitalisation of existing opportunities (Bookman & Bookman, 2007). While, India has managed to enjoy more market share because of the fact that the country had managed to strengthen its capabilities especially in the category of modern healthcare systems and has leveraged its inherent incorporated within the county's traditional healthcare systems (e.g. Siddha, Ayurveda, Naturopathy, Spiritualism and Yoga. Additionally, India has varied tourism destinations (architectural, backwaters, forts, treasures, palaces, springs, hills, jungles and deserts. In short, India geographical conditions and resources are more than enough in catering the needs of tourists in achieving a state of overall well-being. India also has a great edge over other competitor countries as the country is augmented with concentration techniques, mind control, intellectual capital, natural resources, tolerance and cultural diversity (Gupta & Sharma, 2013). Thus it has been contended that India is currently in an advantageous position over many of its major competing countries (Cochrane, 2007).

2.5. Healthcare Tourism in India

India has competitive edge in the healthcare tourism because of certain characteristics: healthcare professional availability, low-cost medical treatment, enhancing popularity of its traditional wellness systems and country's existing reputation for treat of relatively advance healthcare segments (such as organ transplant, cardio-vascular surgery and eye surgery). It had been discovered through the findings of International Passenger Survey that over 2.2% foreign medical tourists visited India for the purpose of obtaining or undergoing healthcare services and medical treatment (Woodside & Martin, 2008). Moreover, the International Passenger Survey had projected that from the sum 2 million non-resident Indian about 10% of which used to come to India with healthcare motive. Therefore, there have been huge number of International tourists (together with non-resident Indians) come to India for undergoing wellness systems: Yoga, Ayurveda and Spiritual Healing. Hence estimated number of travelers who come to India in regard to this category is almost 200,000 on an annual basis (Shanmugam, 2013).

According to Incredible India (2005), it had been estimated that the average spending of International Travelers coming to India is around $2,000 per person. While the calculated overall expenditure incurred by foreign medical tourists is arounf $200 million on per year basis (Fitterling, 2008).

Correspondingly, it has been observed that about 10% of general foreign tourists visit India for pursuing wellness system and used to spend 20% of their aggregate expenditure for healthcare purposes. It has been discovered that the general spending of these travelers reach to $150 annually. By putting all figures together, it has been inclined that India used to generate approximately $600 million from its healthcare tourism industry (Kumar, 2008). And it has been determined that this industry is still growing at fast intensity and is also making significant impact on the country's GDP[2] (Gross Domestic Product)   .

2.6. Initiative in India with respect to Healthcare Tourism

Massive inflow of foreign medical tourists for a broad healthcare service spectrum (ranges from wellness tourism to surgery & rehabilitation) has intended all of the country's stakeholders to focus more on the given industry's unexplored potential; It has been analysed that two major stakeholder: Industry and Government (either state or central governments) are jointing or independently taking initiative with an objective of making India as hot favourite destination for healthcare especially from the perspective of foreign medical tourists (Botterill et al., 2013).

2.6.1.   Industry Initiatives

It has been seen that majority of Indian healthcare centers are developing their medical services along with the patient handling infrastructure according to the world

---

[2] Economic Measure of a country.

class infrastructure standards (Bliss, 2010). The core objective behind these developments is to attract more international medical tourists to India. While the hospitals are also upgrading their technology on consistent basis through the acquisition of state of the art medical equipments. In this regard, they have set-up comprehensive diagnostic centres, world-class blood banks and imaging centres. Relatedly, some hospitals have development separate and special wards (equipped with special information desks[3]) for foreign medical tourists

Alternatively, some hospitals have found it better to operate only in one particular field (ophthalmology, cardiology and dentistry). And few of them have established specialty centers intended on certain areas such as surgery and transplantation. There are also some hospitals who have been organising international conference on frequent basis in the area of their specialities and used to invite medical fraternities belong to different countries so that they would able to showcase Indian skulls in the respective healthcare segments (Kapoor, 2011). It has been believed that such conferences are also instrumental in facilitating the interactions of their specialists which then enhance the process of knowledge transfer.

There are also some hospitals that have created collaboration with both (developing and developed countries). It has been examined that such collaborations are established with other countries' healthcare institutions, hospitals, Government health departments and family welfare which would enable these (Indian) hospitals to participate heavily in healthcare delivery, their patients' treatment and the training of their paramedical & medical professionals (Gautam, 2008). Hence, such collaborations have been facilitating the flow of selected countries' patients to Indian hospitals and the expenses of such treatment would be covered through the national health programmes of respective countries.

It has been identified that there are some hospitals who are undergoing or pursuing the process of constant innovation term of products, facilities and services with the aim of offering better value to their patients and also to remain ahead in the competition. While, some hospitals are concentrating on adopting and utilizing cost effective customer focused technology. However, accreditation and standardization are related strategies followed by major players of Indian Healthcare Tourism

---

[3] Offices where officials are responsible for oragnising and controlling travel requirements, language translation and patients' food & beverages needs.

hospitals. It has been observed that there are increasing number of healthcare institutions that going for obtaining International accreditation of hospitals & clinical laboratories (Conrady & Buck, 2008).

Establishments of Indian healthcare are also looking to adopt aggressive marketing and promotional strategies. In this regard, they used to participate actively in International exhibitions (trade fairs) and International medical symposia. Social communication websites (such as facebook, twitter and Instagram) have also been used in order to promote their services and facilities and also for having direct communication with their existing and potential foreign tourists. Indian healthcare industry has also formed Indian Healthcare Federation (IHCF) with intention of promoting their healthcare industry collectively (Rutherford, 2009).

The approach of telemedicine has also been pursued by many hospitals for the purpose of promoting Indian corporates along with the aspect of providing healthcare services. One more of motive of this promoting concept is to undergo their social obligations of assisting Rural Health Mission which has been formed by the Indian government. While, there are some hospitals who used follow this concept with the purpose of providing distance consulting and treatment advice to their patients located abroad.

2.6.2. Government Initiatives

Government of India's ministries of Health and Family Welfare and Tourism are developing an approach with an intention of giving a strategic push in order to open the country's healthcare sector to medical tourists. The National Accreditation Board for Hospitals have been establishment under the supervision of Indian Quality Council for the hospitals' accreditation. However, Indian government is also examining the policies implicated by other countries for the purpose of Accreditation so that the government would gain knowledge from their experiences and also would support its healthcare tourism industry to go forward (Sharma et al., 2013). Indian government has also taken the initiative of rationalizing the flow of its foreign medical tourists' traffic. At the beginning of 21st Century, medical tourists were used to be granted tourist visa from its missions located abroad.

Because of the fact that tourist visa is non-extendable, non-convertible and valid only for six months period. The medical tourists and their accompanying had many problems during their in India. With the purpose of resolving that problem, Indian government has initiated new visa category named as 'Medical Visa' which could be obtained by medical tourists and their accompanying persons coming to India (Grace, 2007). Additionally, Indian government has set-up fast-track clearance point for the medical tourists at different airports.

Indian Ministry of Communications and Information Technology has established a framework named as IT Infrastructure for Healthcare (ITIH) for the purpose of prescribing accurate standards of every stakeholder with the purpose of integrating healthcare information network in India (Garzone & Catenaccio, 2009). It has been predicted that this initiative would also bring benefits and value to all involved healthcare players and also their users. In relation to the state level, it has been found out that some governments are participating actively in the healthcare expos held abroad. It has been observed that such activities are utilized as a mean for meeting foreign experts belongs to the medical fraternity and then to briefing them about the potential and competence of Indian healthcare industry (Ball et al., 2009).

At state level, it has been observed that there are some initiative that have been taken by the Indian healthcare industry in collaboration with the state governments Kerala has made concentrated efforts in promoting medical tourism with the leverage of Ayurveda in an extensive manner which has outcome in increasing unexpected amount of tourists in this state (Smith & Puczkó, 2009). It has been examined that Kerala Tourism Development Corporation (KTDC) has been promoting Ayurveda since 1990s within the category of medical tourism. The state government of Kerala has also established Ayurveda healthcare centers in multiple hotels. KTDC has also made collaboration with well-known Ayurveda centers so that it would enable the state government in provided authenticated treatment to the foreign tourists coming to Kerala. KTDC has categorized Ayurveda centers in two main categories: Olive Leaf and Green Leaf a kind of grading or accreditation of these centers. With all of these initiatives, Kerala and Ayurveda are seems to appear as each other synonymous. Importantly, it has been illustrated from the current trend that Kerala is appearing as a state of modern healthcare services provider and all of this has been possible with the vital collaborations of private entrepreneurs of healthcare sector and the states' tourism industry (Devashish, 2011).

It has been determined that the state government of Karnataka has been undergoing the process of establishing Bangalore International Health City Corporation which would offer broad range of healthcare treatments and products to the medical tourists (Chillibreeze, 2006). Moreover, the state government has leveraged the state's IT abilities in order to exploit opportunities of healthcare outsourcing services. It has been projected that such leveraging of IT skills would fancy the chance of enhancing the position of state in the emerging healthcare sector with respect to disease coding, medical billing, claims settlement and forms processing.

In regard to Maharashtra state, it has been discovered that the Infrastructure Development and Support Act (MIDAS) has contracted industry status to the tourism activity with the goal of granting all the incentives and benefits that have given to other industries. Correspondingly, the Maharashtra state government in collaboration with the state's healthcare industry has formed Medical Tourism Council of Maharashtra (Hill & Jain, 2011).

The state government of Gujarat has announced distinction medical tourism policy with an objective of formulating integrated medical tourism circuits that would be located within specialty hospitals (Choudhary, 2007).

Section-3: Case Studies

3.1. Case Study on Escorts Heart Institute & Research Centre (EHIRC)

Escorts Heart Institute & Research Centre (EHIRC) was developed in 1988 with the core objective of emerging as India's leading professional healthcare institution. The institution has specialty in tertiary care, oriented more on cardiac care and various range of high quality products and services. Institution is also seems to be consistent with meeting higher customer expectations (Chaudhuri, 2006).

EHIRC has complete medication services (involving 2 heart station, 4 cath labs and 9 operation theatres) with a capacity of over 300 beds. A remarkable attribute of EHIRC is its air ambulance services provision. EHIRC has been offering this services in collaboration with Deccan Aviation named 'Medivac'. Secondary notable feature of EHIRC is its entire range of investigative tests (specifically in the areas of radiology, nuclear medicine, bio-chemistry, microbiology and transfusion medicine). EHIRC's preventive cardiology department has formulated complete monitored exercise, yoga and life style management meditation. Moreover EHIRC is providing premium quality services in the fields of state of art surgical procedures, invasive & non-invasive cardiology and acute care. Prominently, EHIRC is playing major role in early detection, prevention and reversal of heart disease.

EHIRC's marketing strategies incorporate healthcare facilities provision in regard to tourism within and around New Delhi. In order to promote healthcare tourism, EHIRC has developed facilitation centers in Uzbekistan and Bangladesh where its foreign patients could cardiac surgeons and cardiologists through the facilities of video conferencing. EHIRC is contributing actively in the development of India's healthcare indicators through its community outreach programmer designed for the heart diseas programme. With the purpose of strengthening its commitment in regard to heart diseases prevention or early stage diagnosis, EHIRC has started extensive awareness programmes aiming at creating awareness among community about the prevention and control of heart diseases risk factors.

3.2. Case Study on Frontier Lifeline

Frontier Lifeline Private Limited is an International Centre fr Thoracic, Cardiovascular and Vascular diseases. This healthcare centre has advanced infrastructure which permitted it in catering brad of treatment for cardio vascular disorders. The centre has four advanced technology based operation suites that are equipped and designed for performing most complicated cardiac procedures (Gautam, 2008). The distinctive feature of this hospital is that it has two separate intensive care units (ICUs) for adults and children. Another attractive feature of this hospital is that it has appointed additional facilities entirely for its foreign patients for purpose of their convenience. It has been determined that medical tourists from more than 30 countries used to come to this hospital for undergoing different types of medical treatment.

At Frontier Lifeline, the team of surgeons are seeming to be aware of all latest developments taking place in International surgical technology and techniques. This has permitted them to perform most intricate surgeries for acquired and congenital heart diseases. Additionally, Frontier Lifeline is among the list of very few hospitals that are engaged in progressive research on gene therapy, genetically engineered valves and angiogenesis. Frontier Lifeline is aiming for enhancing healthcare quality with the way of streamlining all procedures and formalities beginning from admission process to the discharge. It has been analysed that the hospital has managed in keeping its treatment charges transparent and formulated under economically sustainable package schemes.

3.3. Case Study on Kerala Institute of Medical Sciences (KIMS)

Kerala Institute of Medical Sciences (KIMS) is a multi-specialty hospital which had been commissioned in 2002 with the motive of becoming a hospital based on state of the art infrastructure for healthcare services. It has been observed that KIMS has 35 specialised clinics for the treatment of several procedures (arthritis, adolescence, allergy, anticoagulant, arthscopy, botox, asthma, contact lens, chronic obstructive pulmonary disease, dysphagia, high risk pregnancy management, haematology, immunization, interstitial lung disease, lung cancer detection, low-back ache (Mathew, 2012), KIMS has over 1000 highly skilled, trained and committed medical and para medical staff for handling advanced diagnostic and operational equipments.

Accreditation and Quality assurance are significant strategies pursued by KIMS for the purpose of ensuring world class level treatment at third world prices.

Technology and medical equipments upgradation is seems to be most preferred area of KIMS. KIMS is also pioneer in term of promoting healthcare tourism in association with the government and semi0government institutions. KIMS is also engaged in promoting healthcare tourism by adopting multi-pronged strategies (superior quality in healthcare, adoption & implementation f patient safety norms and clinical standards). It has been inclined that such measures taken by Kerala Institute of Medical Sciences (KIMS) **are** intending its medical tourists to feel comfort with translation, timely procedures, food choices and backed through proper follow-up treatment. Additionally, KIMS is also offering transparent for its foreign medical tourists either for health maintenance schemes or for elective procedures.

3.4. Case Study on Manipal Health Systems

Manipal Health Systems has capacity of more than 5,000 beds, Whereas, it workforce of 5,000 employees and 1,700 consultant doctors has made it as largest healthcare institution of Asia. Currently, Manipal Health Systems has presence in primary, secondary and tertiary healthcare delivery systems. And such delivery systems has intended the hospital to serve more than 100,000 inpatients and over 1 million out patients (Mal, 2010). Manipal Health Systems' dedicated international patient-care centre has capability of handling all special needs of its foreign medical tourists. Manipal Health Systems has based its services on the approach of ensuring provision of smooth & hassle free experience.

Manipal Health Systems has established Telemedicine which thus permit its foreign patients to interact with the specialists at its Banglore hospital. Moreover, Manipal Health Systems has made collaboration with various countries including Mauritius, Tanzania and Gulf Countries. Manipal Health Systems has implicated its telemedicine centre in Mauritius. While, Manipal Health Systems has made collaboration with Tanzanian Ministry of Health for treating more 3,000 high risk patients and in return Manipal Health Systems will receive $5 million. It has been believed that this collaboration deal will allow Manipal Health Systems to pursue more projects of same nature which then would assist it in saving on capital investment in advanced healthcare services.

Manipal Health Systems has also chalked out significant initiative for attracting huge amount of medical tourists from Gulf countries. It has been seen that Manipal Health Systems is intending towards the provision of becoming world class healthcare institution by the way of exploiting state of the art technology in medicine, research and education. It has been believed that such initiatives would allow Manipal Health

Systems to become most successful and admired healthcare systems in Asia.

3.5. Mediciti Healthcare Services

Mediciti Healthcare Services had been established in 1994 and currently the hospital has capacity of around 200 beds. Mediciti Healthcare Services has been has ten super specialties (cardio thoracic surgery, cardiology, gastroenterology, gynecology, nephrology, neuro surgery, neurology, orthopaedic, pulmonology and urology). Mediciti Healthcare Services assume that superior quality of healthcare service delivery is only possible through ethical, sincere and honest healthcare practices (Reisman, 2010), For this purpose, Mediciti Healthcare Services has instituted support system for ensuring and providing high quality patient care and smooth experience to its patients. Mediciti Healthcare Services is seeking for technological advancement by procuring quality & speedy diagnostic surgery facilities. Mediciti Healthcare Services is the first hospital which has introduced Olympus Scope for the treatment of Gastro-entorology. Correspondingly, Mediciti Healthcare Services is in the process of procuring Flag Panel Cathlab and advanced digital cathlab that would be used for the treatment of Cardiology.

Mediciti Healthcare Services is frequently organizing seminars and conferences with the intension of enhancing its global visibility. Mediciti Healthcare Services has also proposed to target foreign medical tourists by providing value added services by making collaboration with tour operators and hotels. Mediciti Healthcare Services has been catering social healthcare by orienting more on rural health, preventive health and health education. Mediciti Healthcare Services is linked up with YSR Foundation with mission of provision of its healthcare services to poor and rural population.

3.6. Findings

By reviewing all above case studies, it has been analysed that there are certain general practices that are being pursued by these healthcare service providers in India. It includes updation and utilisation of advanced technology & medical facilities, consistent healthcare education, research in medical sciences and the approach of skill development. Almost all analysed hospitals are contributing in healthcare development either through telemedicine or through their own set ups in rural areas. However, for the purpose of skill development some studied medical care institutions have been focused more on medical education. Some hospitals has also made collaboration with healthcare service providers or travel facilities as a vital part of their corporate strategies. .

Correspondingly, all analysed hospitals have assigned more value to quality improvement and accreditation. Majority of analysed healthcare institutions have developed separate department for the purpose of catering the needs of their international medical tourists through single window assistance. Specifically, these range of services usually begin from primary information to the all travel related arrangements. Nearly all researched healthcare institutions are in the growing stage domestically as well as internationally. Additionally, EHIRC is considering to expand its operations through locating its facilities abroad. All hospitals are seem to be agreed on price band their major treatment. And it has been predicted that such strategy would assist all of these healthcare institutions in establishing transparency as well as improving the image of Indian healthcare institutions in global market. .

Section-4: Discussion, Conclusion & Recommendations

4.1. Discussion

From the chapters of Literature Review and Case Study, it has been found that there are certain opportunities and threats incorporated within Indian Healthcare Tourism sectors. These two aspects are briefly discussed below:

4.1.1. Opportunities

It has been anticipated that the factor of increasing number of ageing people would put more pressure already over-burdened developed countries' healthcare systems. Relatedly, it would also increase the ratio of uninsured population as well. In short, it has been believed it would be great opportunity for Indian healthcare tourism sector to experience consistent growth with the way of offering high class of medical services at relatively lower price. Alternatively, it has been observed that India has the surplus of skilled professionals in the area of healthcare services and that is the reason there are huge amount Indian that are practicing in developed countries (United States, United Kingdom and Canada). It has been projected that Indian healthcare tourism sector would not have any concern in future in regard to the shortage of skilled professionals in this sector as well.

Multilanguage Skills is looking to be a prominent opportunity for India in relation to the international healthcare tourism field. Indian people are proficient in speaking and understanding English. And it has been forecasted that this aspect would permit Indian healthcare tourism institution to capitalise in the future time period as well. One of the important reason for India for emerging most favourable destination because of its low cost treatment. And this has been found out that it made possible through cost effective measures taken by major players of Indian healthcare tourism sector. Along with the low cost aspect, it has been contended that the success rate of Indian healthcare institutions are also comparable with the standards of developed countries and this would be a significant factor in supporting Indian healthcare hospitals to utilise all given opportunities in a better way.

It has been believed that long waiting time in various would have positive impact on the growing intensity of healthcare care tourism sector especially in regard to the developing countries. Developed countries (like Canada and UK) which intended on providing free healthcare services to their citizens are appearing a major source countries from where significant amount medical tourists have been coming to India for the purpose of obtaining healthcare services. Additionally, it has been inclined that the growth and promotion of healthcare tourism sector would outcome in making positive impact on the development of other medical segments (medical equipments manufacturing, medical diagnostics, telemedicine, hospital administration outsourcing and health insurance). Correspondingly, the growth factor of healthcare tourism would create development opportunities for associated sectors[4] as well.

4.1.2. Challenges

Despite of experiencing massive success in the healthcare tourism at global level, it has been analysed that there are certain challenges that are being faced by the Indian healthcare tourism sector. All of these challenges are described in detail below:

It has been determined that the major challenge which has been faced by the Indian healthcare tourism sector is the bad reputation of India's healthcare standard. And this problem occurred as a reason of disparity existed between Indian rural and urban regions. Second challenge is linked with the less spending of Indian Government on the healthcare initiatives. It has been estimated that health expenditure made by Indian government is only accounts less one fourth of country's overall health expenditure. Relatedly, because of such limitation in public healthcare spending, it has been learnt that Indian private healthcare sector has been playing major role in improving Indian healthcare infrastructure.

Although Indian healthcare tourism sector has gained the benefit of emerging as low cost healthcare destination for foreign medical tourists. But the Indian hospitals that are concentrating on providing exclusive services to its foreign patients, must need to ensure that these low cost medical services are provided in real terms. And this would only be proved through the way of obtaining International accreditation of their existing healthcare facilities. It has been analysed that there still many Indian hospitals that have neglected this aspect which would have negative influence on the existing reputation of Indian healthcare tourism sector. Moreover, it has been inclined that the negative perceptions about India in regard to public hygiene or sanitation standards is a big challenge for the potential growth of Indian healthcare tourism sector.

Indian Human Organs Transplant Act 1994 does not allowed foreigners to avail organs

---

[4] Airline Industry, Hospitality sector and Insurance sector.

from local donors. It has been observed that this challenge has narrow the scope of transplantation tourism in India.

With the booming growth in healthcare tourism sector, it has been analysed that the demand of hotel accommodation is also increasing in India. But it has been observed that the availability of hotel rooms is much lower in India than other countries. Additionally, dual tariff system and the accommodation cost are regarded hindrances to foreign medical tourists coming to India. Therefore, it has been inclined that Indian malpractices law is serving as deferent to Indian healthcare tourism sector. While, it has been believed that better malpractices in India would provide comfort foreign medical tourists and it would also permit these foreign medical tourists to recourse especially in case of complications.

4.1.3. Strategies

In order to exploit certain available opportunity along with the aspect of off-setting all given challengers that have been faced by the Indian healthcare tourism, sectors, there are various strategies that should be adopted by all involved stakeholders at three different levels. These strategies and levels have been listed below:

a) **Policy Level**
- Intending more In-Country Healthcare
- Defining and Enforcing Healthcare Facilities Minimum Standards
- Formulating a Policy based on Composite Healthcare Tourism
- Stimulating Investment in Country's Healthcare Infrastructure

b) **Corporate Level**
- Advancement in Technology
- Creation of Cost Effective Facilities
- Actively contributing in Continuing healthcare education
- Leveraging upon the Potential of Indian Wellness Systems
- Healthcare Sills' Marketing Segmentation
- Great Extent of Public & Private Collaboration

c) **Institution Level**
- Adoption of Patient Centric Approach
- Adhering the Safety Norms of Foreign Patients
- Leveraging Medicine's Traditional Services
- Implementing Intensive Marketing Mix Strategies.

4.2. Conclusion

It has been concluded that Healthcare Tourism and Medical Tourism are interchangeable terms. The concept called as medical tourism is basically from the practice where people belong to developed countries are traveling to the developing countries for the purpose of receiving long range of medical services significantly because of increasing cost of medical services available in their native countries. However, healthcare tourism is described in a broader prospect where the patients are desiring to travel aboard with the motive of overall wellness with any elective or urgent medical procedures. In general, there are two main causes (developed countries' increasing cost of healthcare services and their overburdened healthcare infrastructure) that have resulted in enhancing the demand for healthcare tourism Medical Malpractices Insurance is the major for increasing the healthcare cost in developed countries. Commonly, medical malpractice insurance is considered as major aspect for increasing the cost of medical treatment, widening the delay in the waitlist and also enhancing the movement of medical professionals from one region to another. Hence it has been seen that the increment in the cost of medical treatment also directs towards unaffordable premium in relation to insurance by individuals and thus put large amount of people out from the bracket of health insurance coverage.

India has competitive edge in the healthcare tourism because of certain characteristics: healthcare professional availability, low-cost medical treatment, enhancing popularity of its traditional wellness systems and country's existing reputation for treat of relatively advance healthcare segments (such as organ transplant, cardio-vascular surgery and eye surgery). It has been seen that majority of Indian healthcare centers are developing their medical services along with the patient handling infrastructure according to the world class infrastructure standards. The core objective behind these developments is to attract more international medical tourists to India. While the hospitals are also upgrading their technology on consistent basis through the acquisition of state of the art medical equipments. In this regard, they have set-up comprehensive diagnostic centres, world-class blood banks and imaging centres. Relatedly, some hospitals have development separate and special wards (equipped with special information desks[5]) for foreign medical tourists

---

[5] Offices where officials are responsible for oragnising and controlling travel requirements, language translation and patients' food & beverages needs.

By reviewing all above case studies, it has been analysed that there are certain general practices that are being pursued by these healthcare service providers in India. It includes updation and utilisation of advanced technology & medical facilities, consistent healthcare education, research in medical sciences and the approach of skill development. Almost all analysed hospitals are contributing in healthcare development either through telemedicine or through their own set ups in rural areas. However, for the purpose of skill development some studied medical care institutions have been focused more on medical education. Some hospitals has also made collaboration with healthcare service providers or travel facilities as a vital part of their corporate strategies.

It has been discovered that there are certain opportunities (Increasing cost of healthcare in developed countries, language proficiency of Indians, Indian healthcare institutions' success rate, delay in waiting time, Indian healthcare institutions' success rate and spillover effects) that could be exploited by the Indian medical institutions that are intended on providing medical services to foreign medical tourists. However, it has been determined that Indian medical tourism sector has been some of the challenges (Indian government's low spending on Healthcare sector, lack of International Accreditation, transplantation law, shortage of hotel accommodation and inadequate malpractices law) that could have negative impact on the growth rate of this sector.

4.3. Recommendations

It has been recommended that the strategies currently adopted by major players of Indian medical tourism sector have helped its country to emerge as favourite healthcare destination for foreign medical tourists. It has been analysed that this sector is growing at constant pace however Indian medical tourism sector need some support from its national and state level governments in order to improve image of Indian healthcare sector. Indian Government has taken some of the measures but it has been realised that there are many associated initiatives that should be implemented. And in this way, it would help Indian healthcare institutions to cater more foreign medical tourists.

For the future perspective, one could conduct research on the topic analysis the marketing and human resource strategies that have been adopted by major players of Indian healthcare tourism sector. In this manner, it would help practitioners in identifying the strengths and weaknesses of these strategies.

Section-5: References

- Ball, , Horner, & Nield, , 2009. Contemporary Hospitality and Tourism Management Issues in China and India. London: Routledge.
- Bliss, K.E., 2010. *Key Players in Global Health: How Brazil, Russia, India, China, and South Africa are Influencing the Game*. Washington,D.C: CSIS.
- Bookman, M.Z. & Bookman, K.R., 2007. *Medical Tourism in Developing Countries*. New York: Palgrave Macmillan.
- Botterill, , Pennings, & Mainil, , 2013. *Medical Tourism and Transnational Health Care*. New York: Palgrave Macmillan.
- Chaudhuri, S.K., 2006. *Case studies on competitive strategies*. ICFAI Books.
- Chillibreeze, 2006. *Medical Tourism: A Bangalore Perspective*. Bangalore: Chillibreeze.
- Choudhary, K., 2007. *Globalisation, Governance Reforms and Development in India*. New Delhi: SAGE Publications India.
- Cochrane, J., 2007. *Asian Tourism: Growth and Change*. Oxford: Routledge.
- Connell, J., 2011. *Medical Tourism*. Oxford: CABI.
- Conrady, & Buck, , 2008. *Trends and Issues in Global Tourism*. Berlin: Springer.
- Devashish, D., 2011. *Tourism Marketing*. New Delhi: Dasgupta Devashish.
- Fitterling, L., 2008. *Medical Tourism: A Case Study*. Emporia State University.
- Garzone, & Catenaccio, , 2009. *dentities Across Media and Modes: Discursive Perspectives*. Zurich: Peter Lang.
- Gautam, V., 2008. *HEALTHCARE TOURISM OPPORTUNITIES FOR INDIA*. Mumbai: QUEST PUBLICATIONS.
- George, B.P. & Swamy, G.A., 2012. MEDICAL TOURISM: AN ANALYSIS WITH SPECIAL REFERENCE TO INDIA. *Journal of Hospitality Application and Research (JOHAR)*, pp.1-15.
- Grace, M.A., 2007. *State of the Heart: A Medical Tourist's True Story of Lifesaving Surgery in India*. Oakland: New Harbinger Publications.
- Gupta, & Sharma, , 2013. *Medical Tourism: On the Growth Track in India*. Nrderstedt: GRIN Verlag.

- Hall, C.M., 2013. *Medical Tourism: The Ethics, Regulation, and Marketing of Health Mobility*. Oxon: Routledge.
- Hartwig, R.P. & Wilkinson, C., 2003. *Medical Malpractice Insurance*. Insurance Information Institute.
- Hill, C.W.L. & Jain, A.K., 2011. *International Business: Competing in the Global Marketplace*. New Delhi: Tata McGraw-Hill Education.
- Incredible India, 2005. *India Tourism in 2005*. New Delhi: Incredible India.
- Jagyasi, P., 2011. *Medical Tourism: Research & Survey Report*. www.DrPrem.com.
- James, B.C., 1989. *QUALITY MANAGEMENT FOR HEALTH CARE DELIVERY*. The Hospital Research and Educational Trust.
- Kapoor, S., 2011. *Service Marketing: Concepts & Practices*. New Delhi: Tata McGraw-Hill Education.
- Kumar, B., 2008. *Medical Tourism in India (Management and Promotion)*. New Delhi: Deep & Deep Publications.
- Langenbrunner, J.C., Langenbrunner, & Somanathan, , 2011. *Financing Health Care in East Asia and the Pacific: Best Practices and Remaining Challenges*. Washington,D.C: World Bank Publications World Bank.
- Mal, J., 2010. *Globalisation of Healthcare: Case studies of Medical Tourism in Multi-Specialty Hospitals in India*. Manchester Business School.
- Mathew, B., 2012. *Kerala Tradition & Fascinating Destinations*. Info Kerala Communications Pvt Ltd.
- MIRRER-SINGER, P., 2007. MEDICAL MALPRACTICE OVERSEAS: THE LEGAL UNCERTAINTY SURROUNDING MEDICAL TOURISM. *PHILIP MIRRER-SINGER*, 70(1), pp.212-32.
- Mudur, G., 2004. Hospitals in India woo foreign patients. British Medical Journal, 328. *British Medical Journal*, 1(1), p.328.
- REDDY, S.G., 2013. *MEDICAL TOURISM IN INDIA: AN EXPLORATORY STUDY*. KANSAS STATE UNIVERSITY.
- Reisman, D.A., 2010. *Health Tourism: Social Welfare Through International Trade*. Edward Elgar Publishing.
- Rutherford, A.S., 2009. *India Health: Impact of Medical Tourism Facilities on*

State Health and Economy. Iowa State University.

- Sarkar, A.N., 2009. *Enhancing Global Competitiveness: Advantage India.* New Delhi: I. K. International Pvt Ltd.
- Shah, B.P., 2006. *Asian Hospital and Healthcare Management.* Hyderabad: SPG Media (P) Ltd.
- Shanmugam, K.R., 2013. *Medical Tourism in India: Progress, Opportunities and Challenges.* Chennai: MADRAS SCHOOL OF ECONOMICS.
- Sharma, , Sharma, A. & Tiwari, , 2013. *Changing Face of Medical Tourism in India.* Mumbai: LAP Lambert Academic Publishing.
- Smith, M.K. & Puczkó, , 2009. *Health and Wellness Tourism.* London: Routledge.
- Stolley, K.S. & Watson, , 2012. *Medical Tourism: A Reference Handbook.* ABC-CLIO.
- Vick, L., 2012. *Medical Tourism: Legal Issues.* Michelmores.
- Woodside, A.G. & Martin, , 2008. *Tourism Management: Analysis, Behaviour and Strategy.* Cambridge: CABI.
- Woodward, D., Drager, N., Beaglehole, R. & Li[son, D., 2001. Globalization and Health: A Framework for Analysis and Action. *Bulletin of the World Health Organization*, 79(1), pp. 875-880.